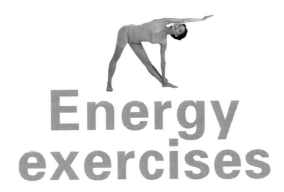

# Energy
# exercises

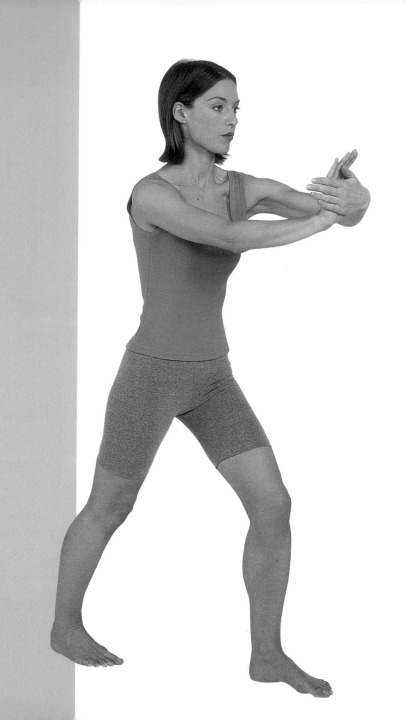

# Energy exercises

Emma Mitchell

CELESTIAL ARTS

BERKELEY TORONTO

For Alex, Amber, and Zac, for whom my energy flows

Celestial Arts
P.O. Box 7123
Berkeley, California 94707
www.tenspeed.com

A Kirsty Melville book

Distributed in Canada by Ten Speed Press Canada.

Design by Rachel Goldsmith
Illustrations by Halli Verrinder
Photography by Matthew Ward

Library of Congress Cataloging-in-Publication Data is on file with
the publisher.
ISBN 0-89087-979-6

First U.S. printing, 2000
Printed in Singapore

Publisher's note
Before following any advice or exercise contained in this book,
it is recommended that you consult your doctor as to its suitability,
especially if you suffer from health problems or special conditions.
The publishers, the author, and the photographer cannot accept
responsibility for any injuries or damage incurred as a result of
following the exercises in this book, or using any of the therapeutic
methods described or mentioned here.

1 2 3 4 5 6 7 8 9 10 — 02 01 00

# Contents

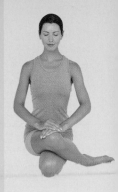

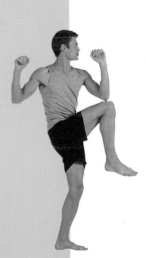

# Introduction

Most cultures and traditions recognize that there is more to a human being than flesh, blood and bones. They acknowledge the existence of a vital energy which reaches beyond the physical – the essence of life. This energy is our most precious possession, and maintaining our energy flow, through exercise and a healthy lifestyle, is the key to realizing our potential, both physically and spiritually.

*Energy Exercises* is a distillation of knowledge gleaned from a range of both Eastern and Western traditions and therapies.

Drawing upon the Eastern concepts of energy, the book introduces disciplines such as T'ai Chi, Qigong and Yoga, suggesting exercises, postures and movements to stimulate and encourage energy flow. It also features exercises based on the Western technique of Kinesiology and on the therapeutic qualities of Egyptian dance.

By practicing the exercises in this book you can experience their energy-boosting benefits for yourself, and improve your overall health and happiness.

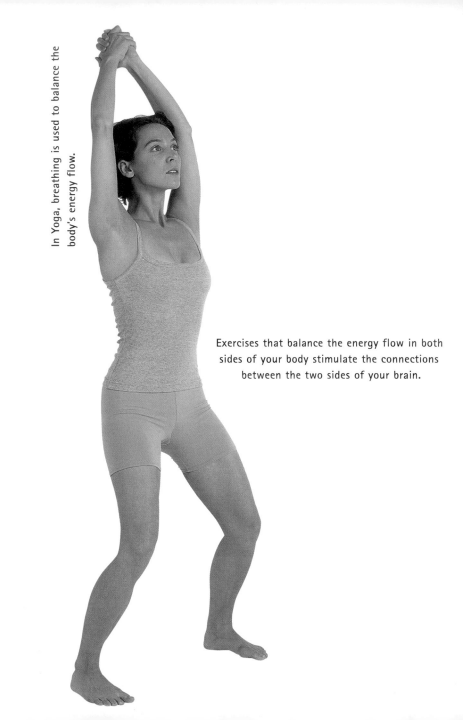

In Yoga, breathing is used to balance the body's energy flow.

Exercises that balance the energy flow in both sides of your body stimulate the connections between the two sides of your brain.

| chapter one |

# *Energy*
# balance

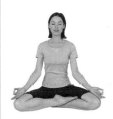

## By stimulating the flow and restoring the natural balance of energy in our bodies, we can vastly improve the quality of our lives.

Energy flows through the body like a river and its tributaries, but often the stresses of Western living act like dams to cause flooding or drought, and disrupt the body's natural, harmonious state.

Imagine that you are able to summon up extra energy or switch off and relax at will. Imagine that your immune system reacts instantly to repel disease, and that you are nurtured with deep, nourishing sleep, and wake up feeling rejuvenated and eager to fulfill the potential of each day. When our body's energy flows freely and in balance, these benefits fall open to us.

# Visualizing energy

**1** Standing with both feet planted firmly on the ground, cross your right leg over your left leg and your right arm over your left arm; now link your fingers together. **2** Keeping your fingers locked, twist your hands under and up, and at the same time press your tongue to the roof of your mouth. Breathe deeply, and visualize energy flowing around your body for one minute. **3** Keeping your tongue pressed into the roof of your mouth, uncross your arms and legs. Stand with your feet apart, bend your arms up and touch fingertips, then breathe deeply for one minute. Repeat the whole sequence, this time crossing your left leg over your right leg and your left arm over your right arm.

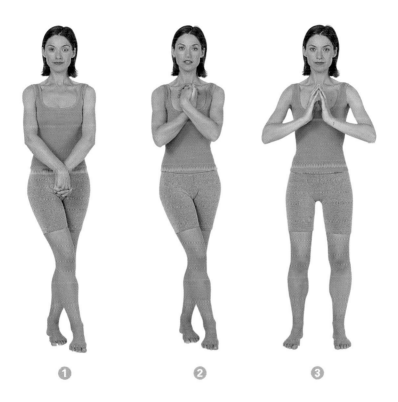

1   2   3

This Kinesiology exercise, known as "Cook's Hook-up", is perfect to do first thing in the morning – it ensures that your energy flow is balanced from the very start of the day.

**Go on! Kick-start your energy!**

Our bodies have evolved so that they produce extra adrenaline (epinephrine) when we are threatened. This makes our hearts pump more blood to our muscles to enable us to fight a predator or run away from danger. Today, we are more likely to face traffic jams than wild animals and, as aggression or escape are no longer appropriate responses, we tend to block the out-flow of excess energy, thus contributing to the build-up of stress.

These exercises (pp.13–15) provide safe, alternative ways to release accumulated tension and re-establish your body's energy balance.

# Fight or flight

the natural energy rush

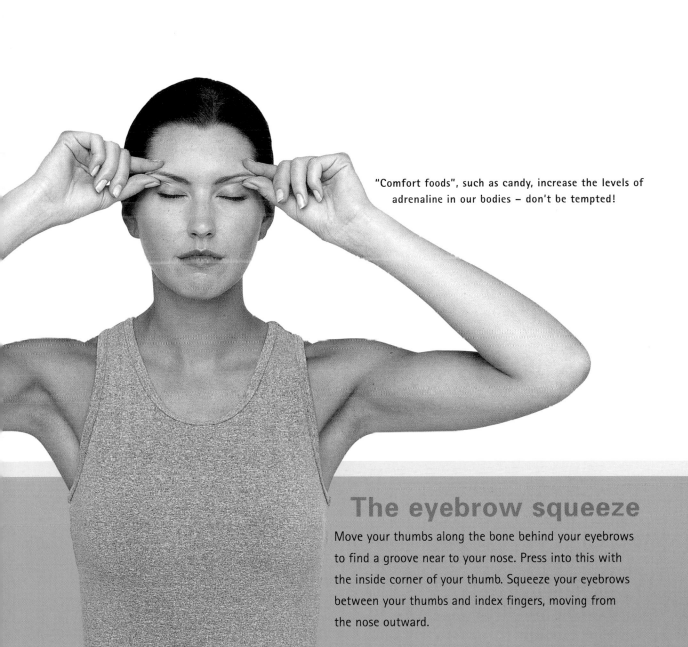

"Comfort foods", such as candy, increase the levels of adrenaline in our bodies – don't be tempted!

## The eyebrow squeeze

Move your thumbs along the bone behind your eyebrows to find a groove near to your nose. Press into this with the inside corner of your thumb. Squeeze your eyebrows between your thumbs and index fingers, moving from the nose outward.

# The wood chopper

**1** Stand, feet shoulders' width apart, knees bent. Clasp your hands together and lift your arms above your head, raising your chest and taking a deep breath. **2** Swing your arms down while exhaling and shouting "Ha!" as loudly as you can. **3** Keep the swing going until you have reached your arms as far through your legs as possible. **4** Swing your arms up again until they are high above your head. Repeat as many times as you feel are necessary to release any excess energy in your system.

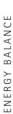

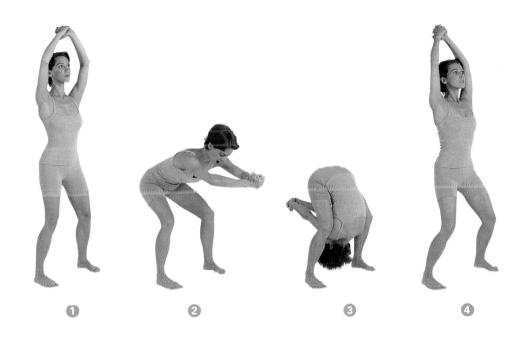

①         ②         ③         ④

This Polarity Therapy exercise releases blocked energy from the solar plexus chakra, which it allowed to build up, can affect your judgment and cause indigestion.

**Polarity Therapy, developed by Dr Randolph Stone (1890–1981), is a form of holistic healing, which treats the mind, body and spirit, and the energy system.**

# Chinese wisdom

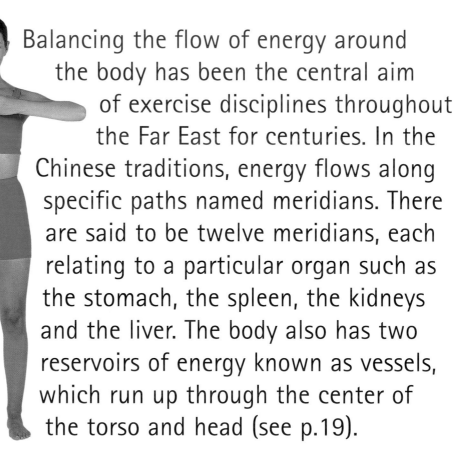

Balancing the flow of energy around the body has been the central aim of exercise disciplines throughout the Far East for centuries. In the Chinese traditions, energy flows along specific paths named meridians. There are said to be twelve meridians, each relating to a particular organ such as the stomach, the spleen, the kidneys and the liver. The body also has two reservoirs of energy known as vessels, which run up through the center of the torso and head (see p.19).

Energy is known as Qi or Chi (pronounced "chee") in China and is created by the tension between two opposing forces, "Yin" and "Yang". The male, Yang energy is represented by the sun, and the female, Yin energy is embodied in the earth.

There are three sources of Qi. We receive Congenital Qi, which is stored in the kidneys, from both parents at conception. It is a barometer of our overall vitality, which can be depleted by stress, lack of sleep and stimulants – dark rings under the eyes are a sign of low Congenital Qi. Nutritive Qi enters the body through the air we breathe and the food we eat. Protective Qi surrounds our bodies. It prevents us suffering from excess cold or heat, and strengthens the immune system. To enjoy good health we need constantly to replenish our Qi and encourage a strong, balanced flow around the body, by practicing energy exercises such as T'ai Chi and Qigong, and by breathing correctly, eating natural foods, drinking fresh water and benefitting from the right amount of sleep.

When we are affected by stress, shock, toxins or emotional problems, the meridians become blocked and this can cause imbalance in and impede the body's energy flow, in turn causing disease. There are specific exercises for removing such blockages (see pp.22–3).

# Rivers of energy

the meridians

Each of our twelve meridians has two channels, one on each side of the body. The meridians form six pairs. One of each pair is a Yin meridian, drawing up energy from the earth. This energy flows up the insides of the legs, up the body, and along the insides of the arms to the fingertips. The six Yang meridians draw Qi down from the sky, and the energy flows from the fingertips to the shoulders, head and body, and down the outsides of the legs.

**Though we cannot see them, the meridians of the body can be measured electrically. Tests have led practitioners to believe that they are located just under the skin.**

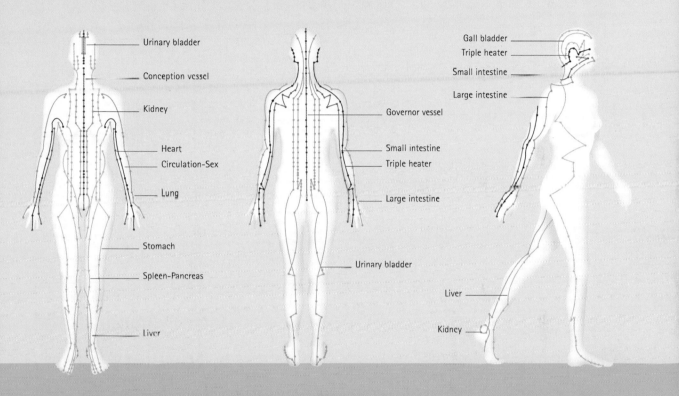

The meridians are all connected. The Qi flows along them in a particular direction and around the body in a continuous cycle (see arrows in the key, right). The Yin meridians are those of the lung, spleen-pancreas, heart, kidney, circulation-sex and liver; the corresponding Yang meridians are those of the large intestine, stomach, small intestine, urinary bladder, triple heater and gall bladder.

Lung→ ● Large intestine→
Stomach→ ● Spleen–Pancreas→
Heart→ ● Small intestine→
Urinary bladder→ ● Kidney→
Circulation-Sex→ ● Triple heater→
Gall bladder→ ● Liver→

Governor vessel ● Conception vessel

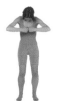

# Achieving and maintaining balance

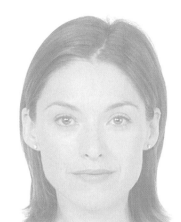

❶ Adopt the Qigong Basic Posture (see p.31). Bring your elbows up and fingers in to the breastbone. ❷ Reach out your arms; keep your shoulders relaxed and imagine wrapping your arms around a huge ball of energy. ❸ Sweep your arms forward, squeezing the "ball"; bring your fingers back to your breastbone and drop your head forward. Repeat 15 times.

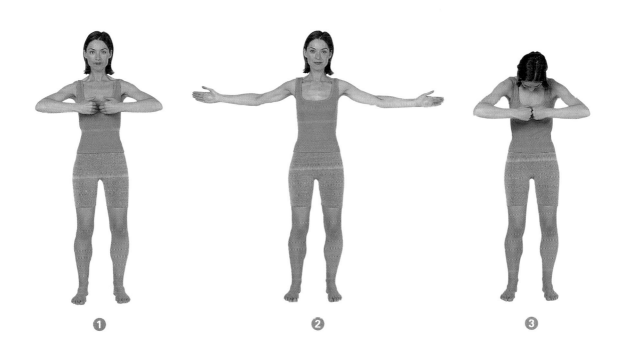

1   2   3

We often throw our bodies out of alignment by carrying a bag (or even our baby) with one arm, or standing with more weight on one leg, or always sleeping on one side. This exercise improves our bodies' symmetry, which opens up the central energy channel and balances energy flow around the whole body.

**Ancient Chinese Daoists believed that a balanced flow of Qi was the key to a long, healthy life.**

# Unblocking the meridians

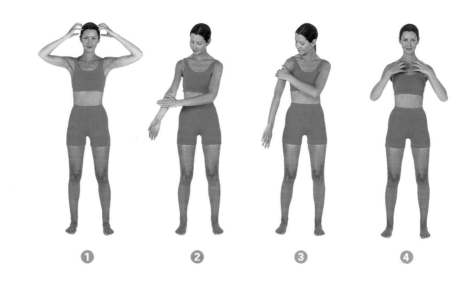

**1** Tap all over your head with your fingertips, then stroke your hair. **2** Brush down the inside of each arm, from armpit to fingertips. **3** Brush up the outsides to the shoulders. **4** Tap your upper chest.

In this Qigong exercise the hands sweep every meridian in the direction of the energy flow. In this way the movement of energy will break through any blockages, restoring balance and increasing vitality.

**Launch into the day with this energy booster – it is especially good for banishing sluggishness in the morning.**

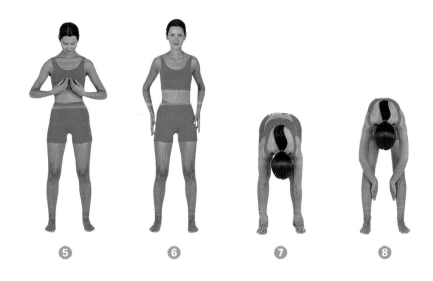

**5** Run your fingertips down your breastbone. **6** Pat your hips and smooth down the outsides of your legs. **7** Pass your hands over your feet. **8** Continue up the insides of the legs. Repeat 10 times.

# Wheels of energy

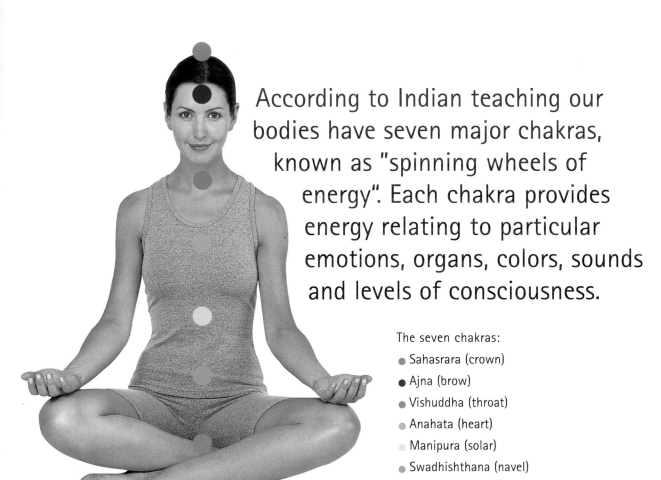

According to Indian teaching our bodies have seven major chakras, known as "spinning wheels of energy". Each chakra provides energy relating to particular emotions, organs, colors, sounds and levels of consciousness.

The seven chakras:
- Sahasrara (crown)
- Ajna (brow)
- Vishuddha (throat)
- Anahata (heart)
- Manipura (solar)
- Swadhishthana (navel)
- Muladhara (root)

The lower chakras generate energy, or *prana*, for the physical body and the pleasures that relate to it, such as eating, drinking and sex. The higher chakras stimulate the emotional and spiritual energy we need for more complex purposes, such as using our intuition, or finding fulfillment and enlightenment.

The seven major chakras are positioned up the midline of the torso and head, from the root chakra at the base of the spine, to the crown chakra at the top of the head. They correspond to important nerve centers in the body, and distribute energy by sending it along a network of 72,000 channels, known as *nadis*.

Energy from the chakras also emanates beyond the physical body to form the aura – a band of shimmering light that surrounds the body in seven layers, each of which has a different color, density and function. The aura is invisible to most people, but those who are able to see it confirm that the layers correspond to those traditionally associated with the chakras. Healers can see and feel the state of a person's health from the colors and vibrations in the electrical field that makes up the aura.

A good way to stimulate the chakras is to practice the holistic discipline of Yoga, which increases all our energy levels: physical, emotional and spiritual.

Like Traditional Chinese Medicine, the Indian practice of Yoga teaches the importance of maintaining a free flow of energy around the body to ensure good health. Yogis advise living in harmony with nature, and balancing energy flow through posture and control of the breath. All Yoga postures form a circuit of energy, and deep, quiet, regular breathing relaxes the body and helps to calm the mind. Yoga can include meditation – cleansing the mind of mental clutter, and stilling thought, often through focusing on a sound or word (known as a mantra), or on a positive reflection.

# The path of Yoga

postures, breathing and meditation

Although there are five types of Yoga, Hatha Yoga (emphasizing postures and movement) is the most widely practiced in the West.

Breathing deeply helps us to absorb more oxygen, which boosts the metabolism and gives the brain better powers of concentration.

# Focus and breath in the half lotus

Sit cross-legged and rest one foot on the opposite calf to take up the half lotus position as shown.
Place the backs of your hands on your knees and touch your thumbs and index fingers together.
Close your eyes or gently focus on the ground. Relax your jaw and touch the roof of your mouth
with your tongue. Imagine your spine rising up effortlessly and the crown of your head reaching
into the sky. Breathe slowly and deeply through your nose, and think of something pleasant, or
repeat one word or phrase with a round, resonating sound such as "happy day", "Ahhh" or "Om".

27

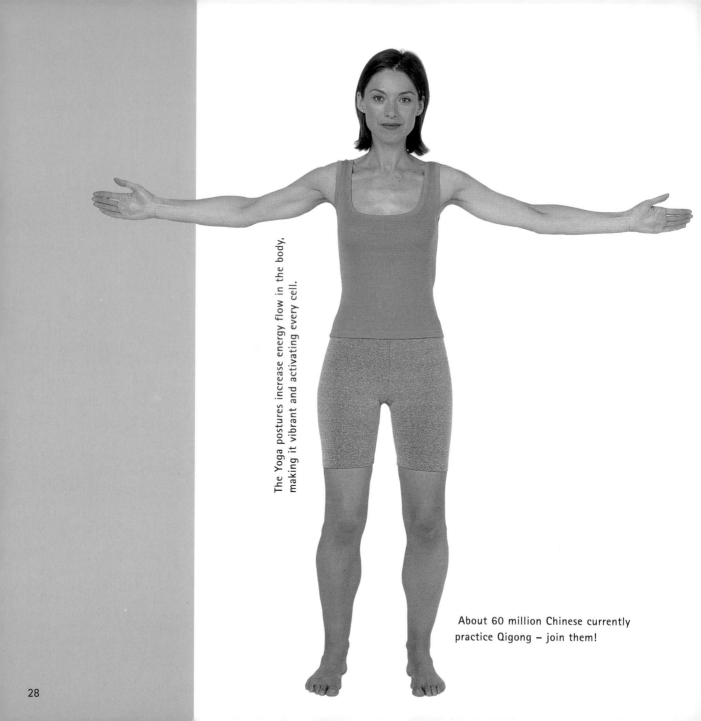

The Yoga postures increase energy flow in the body, making it vibrant and activating every cell.

About 60 million Chinese currently practice Qigong – join them!

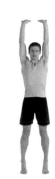

# chapter two

# *Flow better, feel better*

Eastern traditions teach that when our energy flow is strong and healthy we can realize our true potential.

In China and Japan the body is regarded as a microcosm of the universe – by being in tune with the cosmic flow of energy we will gain health, peace of mind and spiritual strength. In India it is believed that we take in vital energy through the breath. This awareness of the body's energy flow is integral to the culture, medicine and spiritual development of many peoples in the East. The following Qigong (Chinese) and Yoga (Indian) exercises increase the body's flow of energy, and promote clear thinking, emotional stability, and happiness, as well as physical fitness.

# Qigong

The ancient Chinese tradition of Qigong has a history stretching back more than 5,000 years. Today it is practiced by millions of Chinese to promote energy flow for health and spiritual wellbeing.

The word Qigong is made up of two Chinese words: *Qi*, meaning energy or vitality, and *gong*, meaning practice. Together they mean "repeated energy work" – the basic (if rather simplified) philosophy behind this Eastern tradition.

Stand, feet parallel, shoulders' width apart. Stretch your feet and splay out your toes. Your knees should be slightly bent and gently eased outward by your thighs. Gently draw up your abdominal muscles and allow your buttocks to sink toward the floor – from the waist down, your body should feel grounded. Lower your shoulders, drop your chin slightly to relax your neck, keeping your head erect as if it is being held from above. Let your arms hang down loosely, as if they were floating slightly outward. You should feel completely balanced and relaxed – if you feel any strain, try to ease it away as you breathe out.

Imagine that you are a tree. Visualize roots growing down from your feet, deep into the earth. You are tapping into the earth's goodness, which you draw up through your roots to nourish you. With each breath, you take in pure, positive energy to stimulate the flow of Qi around your body and, as you exhale, you expel all the negative energy, toxins and anxieties into the earth, where they are absorbed and purified. You feel as if all your cares have melted away. Let your mind rest and feel at peace.

**Qigong is said to be both subtle and internal: subtle because it is non-physical and intangible; internal because it focuses our energy inward.**

# Strengthening the energy flow

**1** Stand, feet shoulders' width apart, knees slightly bent. Elbows out, bring your hands, palms inward, to your chest. **2** Stretch your arms out to the side. **3** Bring them up high above your head. **4** Cradle your skull in your hands. **5** Following the contours of your body, but without your palms actually touching your skin, sweep over your shoulders and, down your chest to your lower ribs. **6** Sweep round to your back so that one hand is over each kidney. **7** Run your palms over your hips and down the outsides of your legs. Sweep round the front of your feet and up your inner calves and thighs, returning to the lower abdomen. Repeat 20 times.

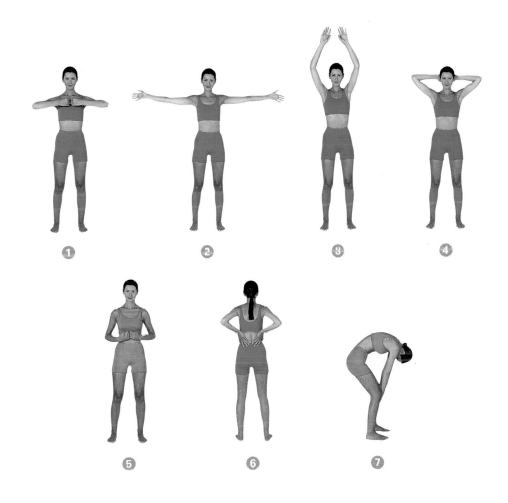

All meridian flow is stimulated by this Qigong movement, but it particularly increases energy flow through the gall bladder (the outsides of the legs, hips and abdomen), the large intestine (the shoulders), and the liver, kidney and spleen-pancreas meridians, which run up the insides of the legs.

**Sweep your body as the mood takes you: whether slow or quick, this exercise will keep your energy flowing strongly.**

# Yoga breathing

**1** Lie flat on your back, arms at your sides. Inhaling deeply, slowly stretch your arms out and up to bring them above your head. **2** As you exhale, stretch your arms out and down. Repeat 5 times. **3** Then, place your palms flat on your ribcage. Breathe in, slowly and deeply, and feel your palms rise as your lungs fill up and your ribcage expands. **4** Exhale, and feel your ribcage contract. Repeat for as long as you wish and sit up slowly when you are done.

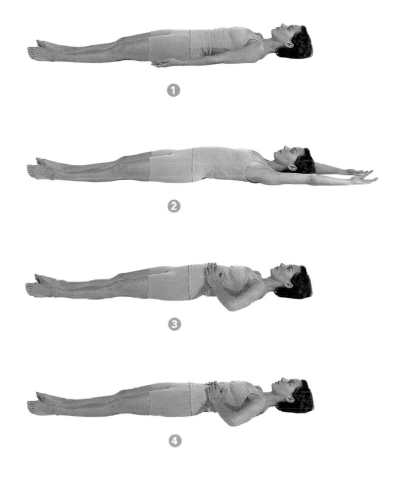

This Yoga exercise expands the chest, opens the lungs and fills the body with life-giving oxygen. It also encourages waste products and toxins to flow out of the body. If you perform it at the end of a stressful day, it will help to establish a good breathing pattern and a positive flow of prana while you sleep.

**Breathe! We can survive for weeks without food and days without water, but only a few minutes without breath.**

# Vertical Yoga stretch

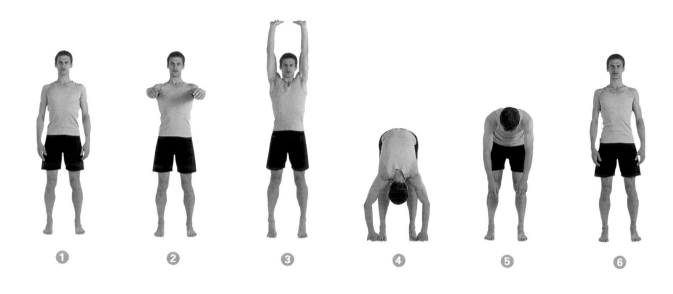

①     ②     ③     ④     ⑤     ⑥

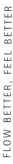

This Yoga exercise is beneficial after a day spent sitting at a desk – it relaxes tense shoulders and strengthens the muscles at each side of the spine. During the exercise the vertebrae are held apart rather then being pushed on top of each other, allowing the cerebral spinal fluid to flow healthily, nourishing the spinal cord and the brain.

**Don't let life get you down – lighten up!**
**This stretch will lift both your body and spirit, and open you out to encourage total energy flow.**

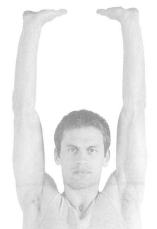

**1** Stand, feet hips' width apart, knees loose, shoulders relaxed. **2** Inhale and reach your arms forward. **3** Stretch your arms upward, go up on your toes and imagine pushing the sky away with your palms. **4** Slowly lower yourself again, finishing with your feet firmly grounded. Exhale and let your upper body flop down like a rag doll. **5** Inhale and gradually straighten up, one vertebra at a time. **6** Finish in the starting position. Repeat 5 times.

# The dog

**1** Rest on all fours, with your hands directly below your shoulders, fingers splayed, knees below your hips, and toes on the floor. **2** Lengthen your spine: push back on your heels and stretch your hands forward as far as you can. **3** Take a deep breath, and as you exhale, push down with your hands while lifting your knees and the fronts of your thighs. Point your buttocks to the sky. Straighten your back and ease your breastbone toward the floor. **4** Bend and lower your knees to return to all fours. **5** Kneel, release your toes, then rest your torso on your thighs, and let your forehead touch the ground. Bring your arms back, palms up and relax your shoulders. Rest, then repeat 5 times.

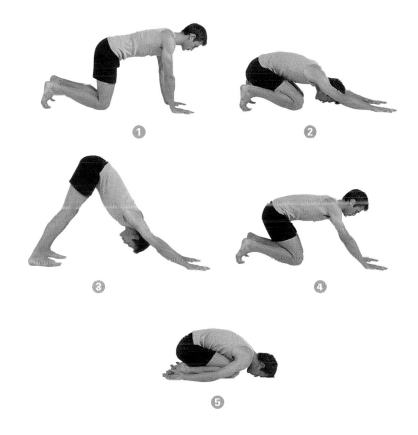

This Yoga exercise opens up the hands, shoulders and hip girdle, allowing energy to flow freely through the body. It warms and invigorates every part and increases blood flow to the head. It also stretches and strengthens the arms and shoulders, and the muscles of the back, buttocks and legs.

**Join our furry, four-legged friends with this morning stretch and wag your tail for the rest of the day!**

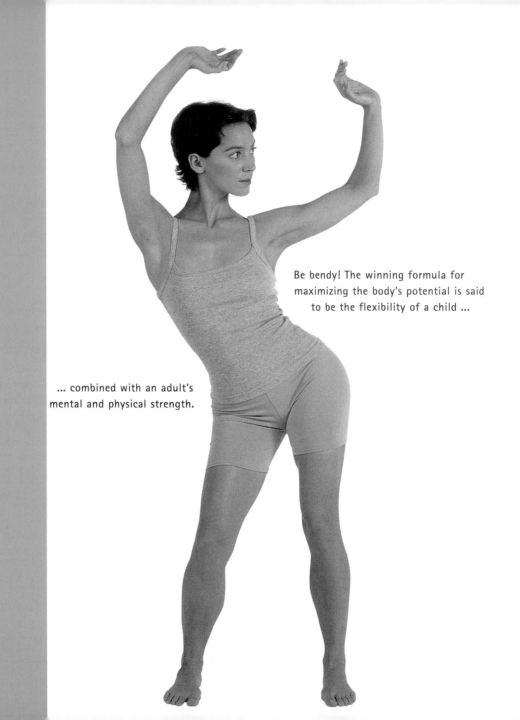

Be bendy! The winning formula for maximizing the body's potential is said to be the flexibility of a child ...

... combined with an adult's mental and physical strength.

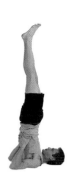

chapter three

# *Flexibility*
# and motion

When we are conscious of our body's
energies, we realize that during movement
we are using energy to create more energy.

In the West the idea of exercise conjures up images of activities

such as high-impact aerobics or jogging. Such strenuous workouts

can impose stress on the body's joints and cardio-vascular system.

As a result, gentler types of exercise such as Yoga, Qigong and

T'ai Chi, which involve the use of static or slow-moving postures,

and require mental as well as physical discipline, are gaining in

popularity. Traditions such as these stimulate energy flow and make

our movements more fluid as well as improving our overall fitness

– without all the huffing, puffing and exhaustion.

# The waist swing

Much of the enjoyment in this T'ai Chi exercise stems from
the graceful, rhythmical movement that increases energy flow.
It relaxes the upper body and calms the mind while toning the
abdominal muscles and massaging the internal organs.

**Swing away stress! This exercise will loosen your shoulders and trim your waist.**

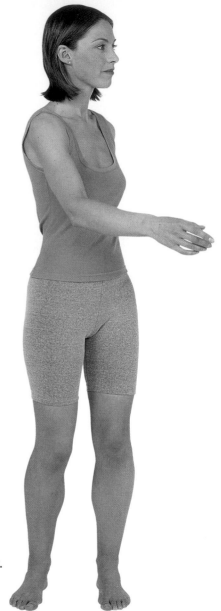

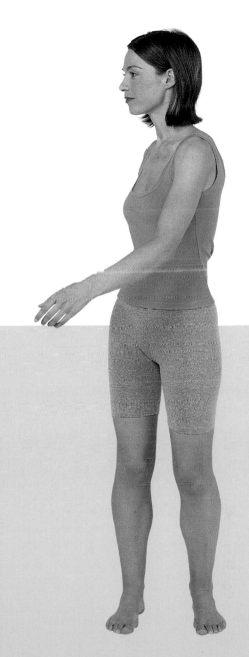

**1** Stand, feet hips' width apart and flat on the ground, knees loose. Keeping the upper body relaxed and the arms floppy, thrust your right hipbone forward and your left hipbone back. **2** Return the swing by pushing your left hipbone forward and your right hipbone back. The twisting motion encourages the shoulders to follow and the arms to swing of their own accord. Concentrate on the hip motion and keep the upper body fluid. Continue until you feel warm and relaxed.

# Pushing and pulling

**1** Stand, feet shoulders' width apart. Inhale, raising your left elbow upward and parallel to the ground, the palm of your hand facing your chest. Raise your right forearm vertically, palm facing forward. Put your palms together. **2** Step forward with your left foot, pressing your right hand against the left, pushing the left hand forward beyond your foot as you exhale. **3** Use your left hand to pull the right one back. Inhale and bring your weight back onto your right foot. **4** Stand, feet parallel, shoulders' width apart. Elbows bent, open your arms with your palms facing forward and exhale. Repeat the whole sequence slowly, 5 times. Swap over to the other side.

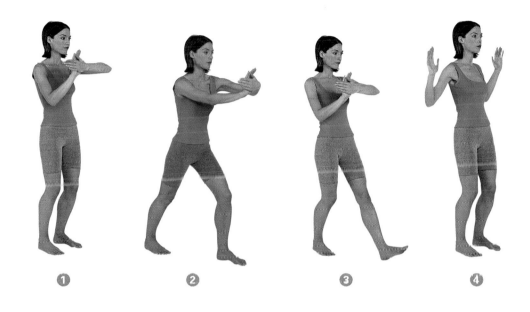

This T'ai Chi exercise promotes the sensitive, flowing and reciprocal motion of energies between the hands. It encourages awareness of the interplay between the opposing yet complementary forces of Yin and Yang (for example, through pushing and pulling, controlling and yielding, giving and receiving) and it helps to restore balance between the two forces.

**Practitioners of T'ai Chi often benefit from a high level of flexibility well into old age – the gentle movements mean that the exercises can be done by anyone, at any time of life.**

# Movement to strengthen the legs

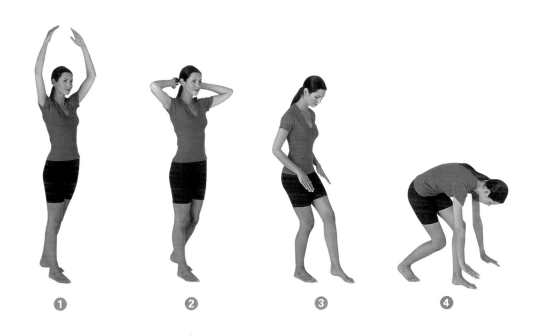

① ② ③ ④

This Qigong walking exercise grounds the body's energy, promoting a good flow. It tones the muscles in the legs, shoulders and arms, and encourages increased flexibility and coordination.

**According to the principles of Qigong, each time we place a foot on the ground when we walk, we are reconnecting with the vital energies of the earth.**

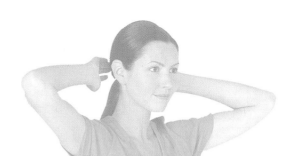

**1** Step forward, put your weight on your right foot, your arms curved above your head. **2** As you begin to move your left foot forward, put your hands behind your head. **3** Sweep your hands over your shoulders and down to hip level as you move your left foot in front of your right and transfer weight onto it. **4** Lean forward at the waist, bend your knees and move your hands as far as you can toward the floor. Repeat 10 times, then swap legs.

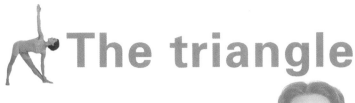 # The triangle

**1** Stand with your feet wide apart. Inhale. Raise and stretch your arms out to the side. **2** Turn your left leg out 90 degrees and push your right heel slightly out to the right. Exhale. **3** Inhale. Stretch your left hand down to hold your left ankle and your right hand straight up. **4** Exhale. Bring your right hand down past your right ear and stretch it out to the left. Inhale. Stand up, arms outstretched. **5** Lower your arms, and point your feet forward. Repeat on the other side.

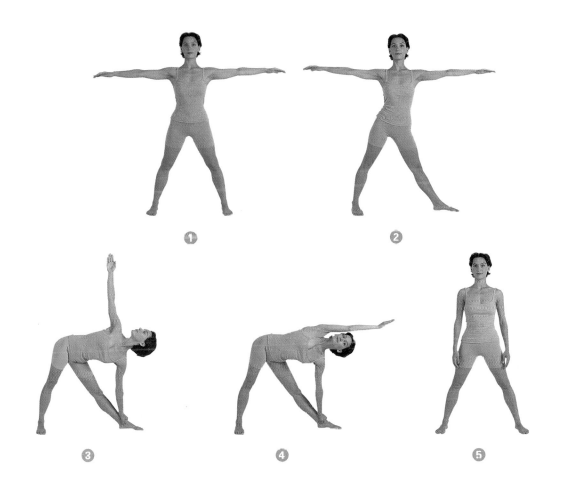

This Yoga pose opens up the hip and shoulder girdles to allow the free movement of energy, and helps to trim the waist, making it more supple.

**For maximum benefit take your time and do this exercise slowly – it creates a really satisfying stretch.**

# The shoulder stand

**1** Lie flat on your back. **2** Place the palms of your hands on the floor, inhale, tighten your stomach, and raise your legs straight up (if this strains your back, bend your knees). **3** Exhale, and continue to swing your legs above your head, lifting your pelvis, and putting your hands on your back. **4** Raise your legs toward the sky and push up onto your shoulders, supporting your back with your hands. Breathe deeply. **5** Bend at the hips and slowly lower your toes to the ground behind your head, drawing up the hips and fronts of the thighs, stretching the backs of the legs. **6** Lift your feet, put your palms flat on the floor, and unroll your back, one vertebra at a time. If you find it easier, roll down with bent knees.

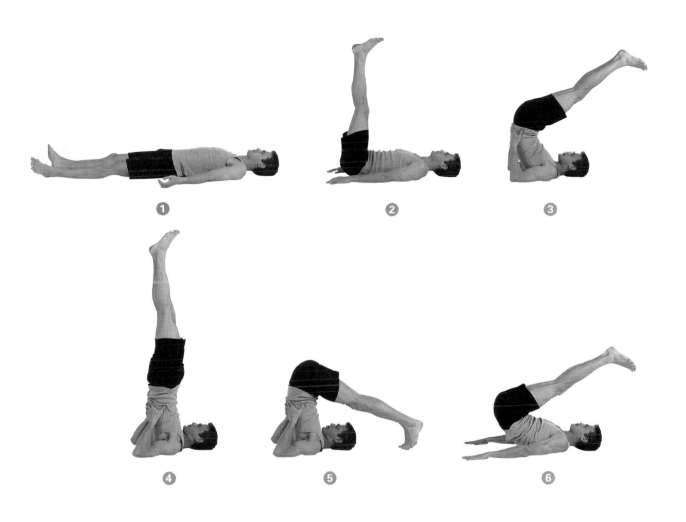

This Yoga exercise tones the whole body and encourages energy flow to the thyroid and parathyroid glands in the neck, but you are advised not to attempt it if you are pregnant, menstruating or suffer from back problems.

**The Fish (pp.52–3) is the counterpose to the Shoulder Stand – turn the page and do the Fish now!**

# The fish

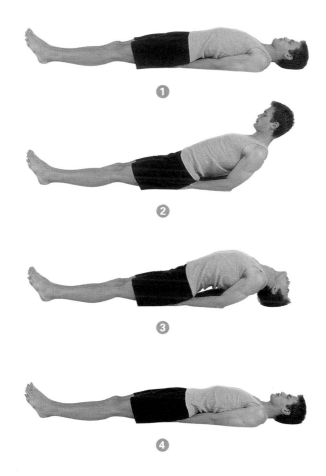

1

2

3

4

This Yoga exercise unblocks energy in the lung, stomach and spleen meridians. It also increases suppleness in the cervical and lumbar muscles in the back, as well as in the shoulder muscles.

**This exercise is called the Fish because it trains the lungs to fill up with air, improving our ability to float in water.**

**1** Lie flat on your back – hands under your bottom, palms facing down, arms straight. Squeeze your shoulder blades together. **2** Inhale and raise your upper body onto your elbows so that you are sitting on your hands, looking at your feet. **3** Exhaling, and keeping your elbows close together, arch your back and rest the top of your head on the ground. Breathe deeply. **4** Release your head, and lower yourself onto the floor so that you are lying flat on your back again.

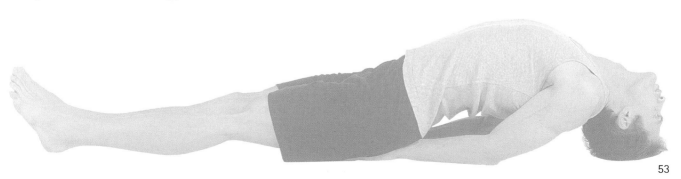

# Egyptian figures of eight

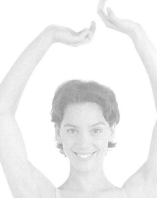

**1** Stand, feet a little more than hips' width apart, firmly on the ground. **2** Keeping your knees slightly bent, move your right hip forward. **3** Push your right hip out to the side and then back, in a smooth circular motion. **4** Without hesitating, move your left hip forward. **5** Push your left hip out to the side and then back. Repeat, leading with alternate hips as if you are outlining a figure of eight. Maintain a rhythm, focusing on fluidly moving your hips while keeping your spine upright. Move your arms in the air to improve balance and add elegance.

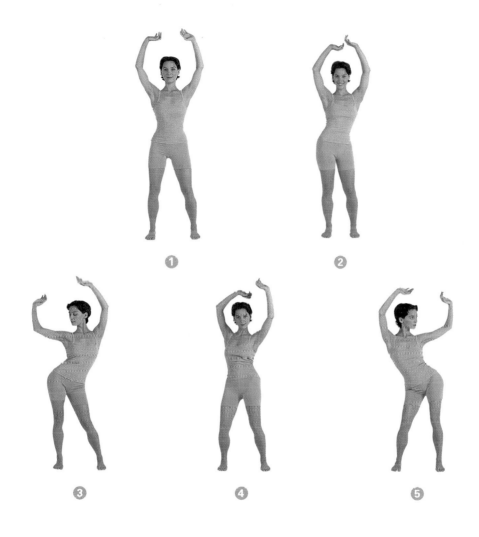

In Egyptian (or belly) dancing, the hips and abdomen move vigorously, leading the rest of the body, while the feet stay still – in this way the dancer maintains a connection with earth energies. Belly dancing tones the waist and hip areas and increases their flexibility. It also helps to heal pelvic, urinary, gynecological and digestive disorders.

**"As long as there is life, there will be dance."** (Margaret N. H. Doubler)

55

# Egyptian hip drops

1 Stand with your feet hips' width apart, your right foot slightly forward. Keep your back and shoulders relaxed. Bend your left knee a little and raise your right heel, keeping the ball of your foot and your toes firmly on the ground. 2 Using your toes to push up, lift your right hip. 3 Bring the right hip forward and then lower it. Allow your arms, held above your head, to flow with the hip movement. 4 Sweep your right hip in a circle, from the front to the side and then back. Repeat Steps 2–4. Continue this sweeping motion for as long as you wish in a rhythmical and smooth movement. Repeat with your left hip for the same amount of time.

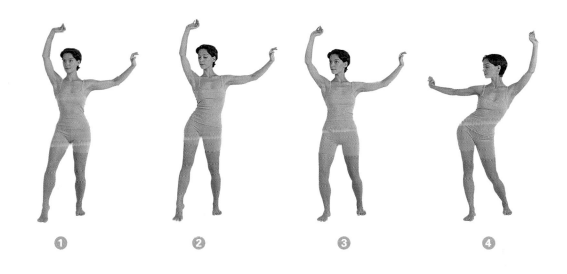

In this Egyptian dance exercise, energy flow is improved in the kidney, liver, urinary bladder, gall bladder, stomach and spleen-pancreas meridians, all of which pass through the pelvic area. Hip drops tone the abdominal, buttock and leg muscles, as well as greatly improving pelvic health and flexibility.

**Dancing is healthy, therapeutic and enjoyable because it promotes flexibility in both body and mind – to dance well we need let go and allow our energy to flow.**

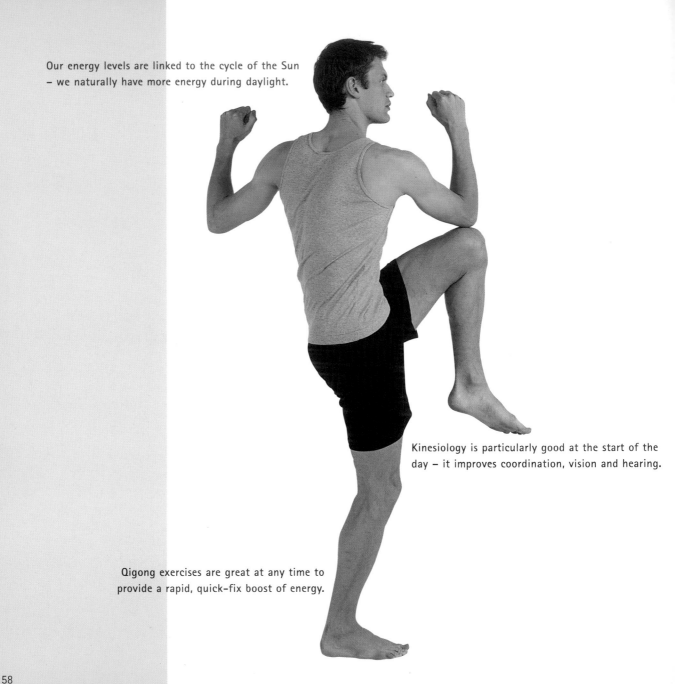

Our energy levels are linked to the cycle of the Sun – we naturally have more energy during daylight.

Kinesiology is particularly good at the start of the day – it improves coordination, vision and hearing.

Qigong exercises are great at any time to provide a rapid, quick-fix boost of energy.

# chapter four

# *Energize* your day

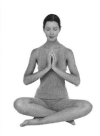

## Understanding the ebb and flow of our energy levels through the day is important for living life to the full.

We all have different body clocks: some people feel sluggish and
find it hard to function first thing in the morning; many have a dip
in energy after lunch; and most of us feel drained at the end of a
busy day. By learning to recognize and anticipate the fluctuations
in our energy levels we can take steps to replenish our reserves
to meet particular challenges at different times in our schedule.
In this chapter there are exercises to improve our energy levels
when we rise, after lunch and in the evening, as well as others that
can quickly boost our energy flow whenever we need vitality most.

# The five-finger fix

**1** Rest the tips of the thumb and four fingers of your left hand over your navel. Place the thumb and index finger of your right hand just below your collarbones. Wiggle all your fingers for 10 seconds to energize the meridians. **2** Keeping your left hand over your navel, place your right index finger on the middle of your top lip and your thumb on the middle of your lower lip, and rub these points for 10 seconds. **3** Place your right hand flat on the base of your spine and massage this spot for 10 seconds while still keeping your left hand over your navel. Repeat with your right hand over your navel and your left hand in the three positions.

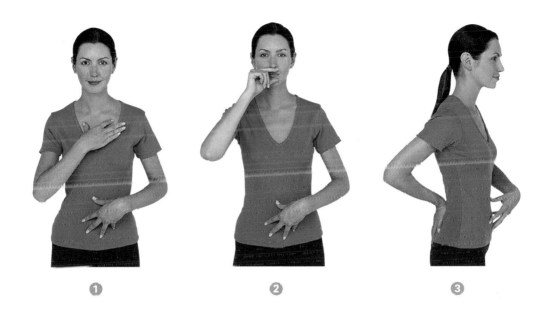

| ① | ② | ③ |

Massaging the two points below the collarbones helps to balance the energy flow in the kidney meridian. The fingers placed around the navel stimulate the flow of all the meridians in the navel area. The index finger and thumb placed on the lips connect the two energy reservoirs – the Governor and Conception vessels. The different actions of the two hands, and the points they massage, encourage the flow of electrical energy through the brain.

**If you wake up feeling "out of sorts", Kinesiology will point your energy back in the right direction.**

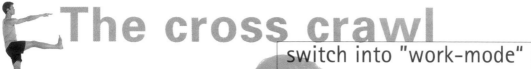

# The cross crawl

**1** Lift one knee and swing the opposite arm so that the elbow touches the knee. **2** Lift the other knee and opposite arm in the same way. Looking at a plain wall, march like this 10 times, on the spot. Continue for another 10 marches, this time rolling your eyes widely in a clockwise movement. Repeat the sequence, this time rolling your eyes counter-clockwise. Now march another 10 times, moving your eyes in a large figure of eight. **3** Raise your right arm and right leg simultaneously 10 times, while following the above sequence of eye movements. Now raise your left arm and left leg, and march 10 times, repeating the eye movements once more. Finish by repeating Steps 1 and 2.

ENERGIZE YOUR DAY

62

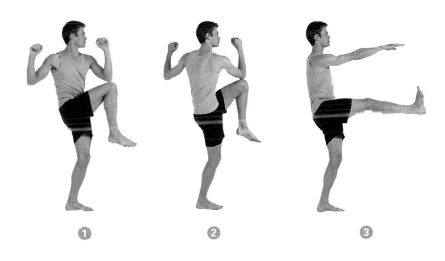

1  2  3

Kinesiology exercises are specifically designed to exercise the brain as well as the body. They improve the connections between the right and lcft hemispheres of the brain by coordinating movements between the two halves of the body. They are beneficial for everyone, but particularly for people with learning difficulties and dyslexia.

**This exercise is based on, and named after, the crawling movements of babies.**

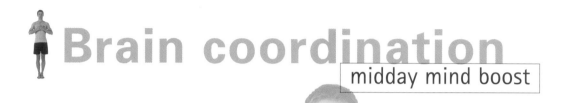

# Brain coordination

**1** Stand, feet together, eyes closed, with your arms at shoulder height out to the sides, palms forward. **2** Slowly bring your arms together until your palms meet – keep trying if this does not happen first time – it's more difficult than you might think. Link your fingers and imagine that you are joining the two sides of your brain. **3** Bring your hands in to your chest as if you are drawing in your whole self. Rest with one hand on top of the other. **4** Relax, hands by your sides, eyes closed, and enjoy the calm, satisfied feeling of your brain being in balance.

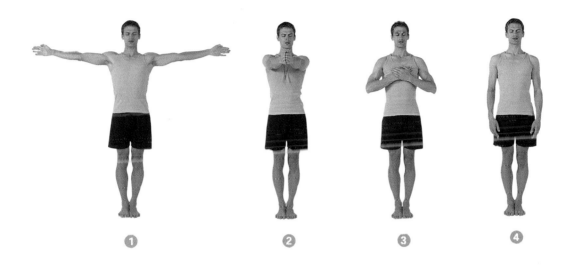

This Kinesiology exercise simultaneously stimulates both hemispheres of the brain so that you think and move in a more coordinated way. It also helps to calm and balance the emotions by integrating confused and conflicting thoughts.

**Try this in your lunch hour – get your colleagues to join in too.**

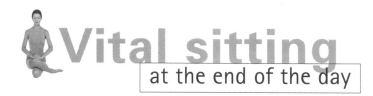

# Vital sitting

## at the end of the day

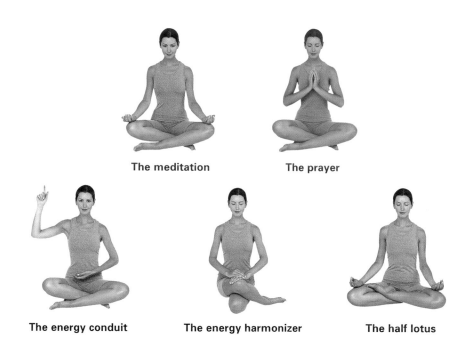

The meditation           The prayer

The energy conduit       The energy harmonizer       The half lotus

The above Qigong and Yoga sitting postures open out the hip and shoulder
girdles, increasing energy flow up the spine. Spend 5 minutes practicing one of
them at the end of the day – close your eyes, breathe deeply and relax.

**In sitting postures, when the hands are in an open position
they receive energy; when they are held close to the body they conduct energy inward.**

**The meditation**  Sit cross-legged, keeping your spine straight (but not strained) and rest the backs of your hands on your knees.

**The prayer**  Touch the tips of your fingers and the heels of your hands together in a prayer position to energize and nourish the heart chakra.

**The energy conduit**  Point one index finger skyward to draw down Qi, your wrist facing forward. Cup your other palm horizontally in front of your navel.

**The energy harmonizer**  Sit on one heel with your upper leg crossed as far as possible over the lower leg, your hands on top of each other on your knee.

**The half lotus**  Sit cross-legged and bring one foot up onto the opposite calf. Place your hands on your knees, keeping the palms open.

# Sensing the energy

**1** Stand, feet shoulders' width apart, knees slightly bent, arms by your sides. **2** Bring your hands in front of your abdomen, palms facing inward. Spend 2 minutes visualizing a ball of energy emanating from your abdomen, filling your hands. **3** Slowly, move your hands apart and imagine the ball of energy growing between them. Keep this position for 1 minute. **4** Now visualize the ball of energy contracting, as it pulls your hands in toward each other. Repeat several times until you can feel the energy expand and contract. **5** Draw your hands in toward your abdomen and imagine the ball of energy contracting back inside into a small spark. Wiggle your hands and shake your fingers.

ENERGIZE YOUR DAY

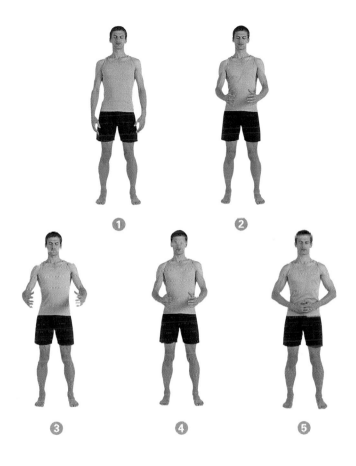

① ② ③ ④ ⑤

This Qigong exercise can give you an energy boost at any time of the day. It helps to increase the flow in the energy center known as the lower dantien, which is located deep in the abdomen. According to Chinese tradition, the lower dantien is the seat of our being and the source of our vitality.

**You will know when you succeed in feeling the energy between your hands – they will tingle or warm up.**

# Energy first-aid

quick-fix tips

Pressing the acupoints encourages the body to maintain its natural energy equilibrium and regulates the energy flow. The following acupressure exercises provide quick-fix self-help to restore the balance in your body.

**Governor Vessel 26** Located a third of the way down the groove in the middle of the upper lip. To make you more alert, or to relieve feelings of faintness, press this point 3 times with your index finger, for 7–10 seconds each.

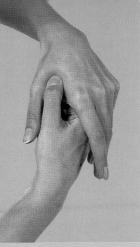

**Large Intestine 4** Found in the fleshy web between the thumb and the index finger. Stimulating the energy flow in this meridian helps to treat diarrhea, rashes and toothache. Press this acupoint 3 times, on both hands, for 10–15 seconds each. It is not advisable to press this point on a pregnant woman.

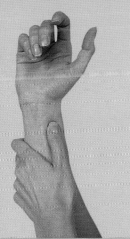

**Lung 7** Located on the forearm, 1¹/₂" below the wrist fold, on the same side as the thumb, in the hollow behind the wrist bone. Pressing this acupoint helps to increase the energy flow to the lungs to combat respiratory problems, common colds and headaches. Press hard with your thumb 3 times, on both wrists, for 7–10 seconds each.

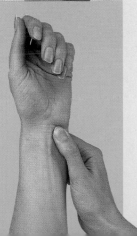

**Heart 7** Found down below the little finger, on the inside of the wrist, just behind the wrist crease. Stimulating this acupoint helps to counteract irritability and to treat insomnia. Support your wrist with the fingers of your other hand, then press this point 3 times, on both wrists, for 7–10 seconds each.

# Index

ACKNOWLEDGMENTS

The publisher would like to
thank models Helen Brumby,
Tim Cummins, Caroline Long
and Kerry Norton, and
make-up artist/hairdresser
Evelynne Stoikou.